GYMST⬦NES FACT⬦RY

KNOW YOUR WORTH.

SELF
DEVELOPMENT
JOURNAL

BY
HEIRESS BRADFORD

AMETHYST
CALM · PEACE · STABILITY

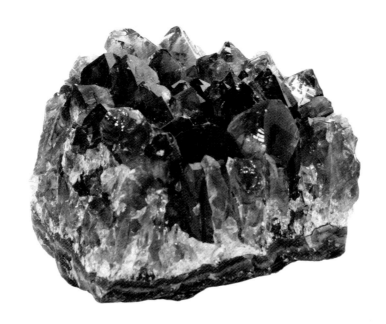

IN THIS JOURNAL
YOU WILL FIND 12-WEEKS OF MOTIVATIONALLY
THEMED SECTIONS THAT GUIDE YOU THROUGH OUR
SHINE© HOLISTIC LIFESTYLE SYSTEM.

SELF-ESTEEM · HEALTH-CONSCIOUS · INTELLECT-DEVELOPMENT
NUTRITIONAL-VALUE · EXERCISE-PRACTICE

BE HONEST AND KIND WITH YOURSELF ON THIS JOURNEY.
THE DECISION TO CHANGE YOUR LIFE IS MAJOR;
NO MATTER HOW MINOR THE ADJUSTMENT.
TRUST YOUR PROCESS!
IT'S YOUR TIME TO SHINE©!

SELF-ESTEEM

HOW DO YOU VIEW
YOURSELF?

WHAT ARE YOUR MOST
POSITIVE TRAITS?

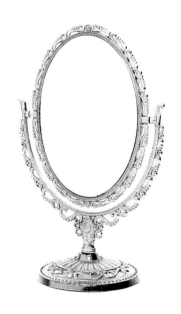

HEALTH-CONSCIOUS

IN GENERAL, MY HEALTH IS BEST
DESCRIBED AS:

SOME THINGS I WOULD LIKE TO
IMPROVE ARE:

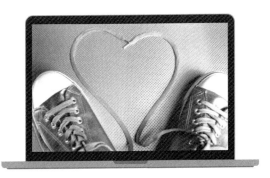

REST
&
RECREATION

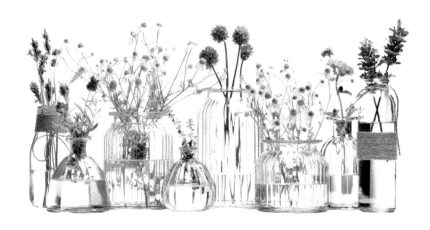

INTELLECT-DEVELOPMENT

```
N  H  E  M  A  T  I  T  E  I  U  I  P  P  L  G
E  L  V  L  O  E  Z  E  X  T  F  D  H  Q  H  A
G  I  R  Y  W  S  Q  A  M  E  T  H  Y  S  T  R
Z  Z  V  M  B  Y  X  R  X  W  E  E  Z  Z  E  N
B  H  G  F  U  W  S  D  H  T  N  E  R  Z  T  E
L  U  A  P  R  A  N  T  A  O  T  R  T  X  M  T
O  X  R  N  O  O  N  G  T  I  N  K  W  J  M  O
O  D  X  K  M  H  A  S  N  I  D  X  V  F  A  A
D  L  D  A  S  E  D  O  U  M  Q  S  E  R  G  B
S  X  I  A  R  L  Z  E  R  W  T  U  W  G  D  G
T  D  H  I  O  A  V  I  K  I  T  D  V  I  U  I
O  P  F  G  M  C  N  C  B  O  X  P  B  B  I  A
N  U  G  A  I  J  T  V  L  C  V  I  T  T  K  R
E  Z  D  L  Y  F  O  H  F  B  V  T  K  G  N  O
H  H  Q  M  T  U  W  I  E  M  E  R  A  L  D  X
X  L  A  P  I  S  L  A  Z  U  L  I  Q  Y  R  Y
```

- ~~Garnet~~
- ~~Diamond~~
- ~~Emerald~~
- ~~Amethyst~~
- ~~Hematite~~
- ~~Amazonite~~
- ~~Fire Agate~~
- ~~Goldstone~~
- ~~Bloodstone~~
- ~~Lapis Lazuli~~

CRYSTALS

NUTRITIONAL-VALUE

INGREDIENTS

3 TABLESPOONS OF
VANILLA PROTEIN
POWDER
1/2 CUP OF FROZEN
BLUEBERRIES
1/4 - 1/2 TEASPOON
OF MAPLE EXTRACT
1/4 TEASPOON OF
VANILLA EXTRACT
2 TEASPOONS OF
FLAXSEED MEAL
PREFERRED
SWEETENER
10-15 MEDIUM ICE
CUBES
1/4 CUP OF WATER

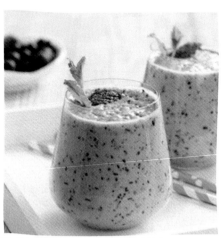

DELICIOUS BLUEBERRY SMOOTHIE

DESCRIPTION
THIS SMOOTHIE. IS LOADED WITH PROTEIN
PREP/TOTAL TIME: 5 MINUTES
SERVINGS: 2

INSTRUCTIONS
1. TRANSFER THE INGREDIENTS INTO A BLENDER AND
BLEND UNTIL WELL MIXED. YOU CAN THICKEN BY ADDING
MORE ICE OR MORE LIQUID BY ADDING MORE WATER.
2. SERVE.

NUTRITION FACTS
PER SERVING
CALORIES: 230
FAT: 5G
CARBOHYDRATES:
18G
PROTEIN: 27.5G

EXERCISE-PRACTICE

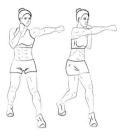

EXPLOSIVE PUNCHES!
1: STANDING WITH YOUR FEET HIP-WIDTH
APART WITH YOUR ARMS BENT IN FRONT OF
YOU AT CHIN LEVEL, MAKE TWO FISTS
2: SWIVEL YOUR RIGHT HIP FRONTWARD WHILE
ROTATING YOUR REAR FOOT SO THAT ONLY
YOUR HEEL COMES OFF OF THE GROUND
3: KEEPING YOUR ELBOWS TUCKED THROW
FAST FORWARD PUNCHES ALTERNATING SIDES

SQUAT-HOLD-PUNCH!
1: STANDING WITH YOUR FEET HIP-
WIDTH APART WITH YOUR ARMS BENT IN
FRONT OF YOU AT CHIN LEVEL, MAKE
TWO FISTS
2: LOWER INTO A COMFORTABLE SQUAT
POSITION AND HOLD IT, ENGAGE YOUR
ABS AND SQUEEZE YOUR SHOULDER
BLADES TOGETHER
3: BEGIN THROWING RAPID PUNCHES
ALTERNATING ARMS

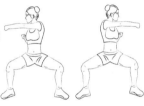

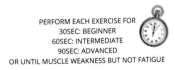

SEATED PUNCHES!
1: STARTING IN A SEATED UPRIGHT POSITION
KEEP YOUR SHOULDERS BACK AND YOUR CORE
FULLY ENGAGED
2: LIFT YOUR FISTS TO EYE LEVEL AND BEGIN
ALTERNATING PUNCHES BE SURE TO FULLY
EXTENDING YOUR ARM
3: RESET TO STARTING POSITION AND REPEAT

PERFORM EACH EXERCISE FOR
30SEC: BEGINNER
60SEC: INTERMEDIATE
90SEC: ADVANCED
OR UNTIL MUSCLE WEAKNESS BUT NOT FATIGUE

REFLECT
&
RELEASE

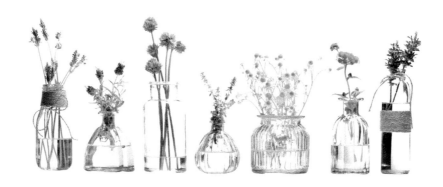

OPAL
CREATIVITY · HOPE · PURITY

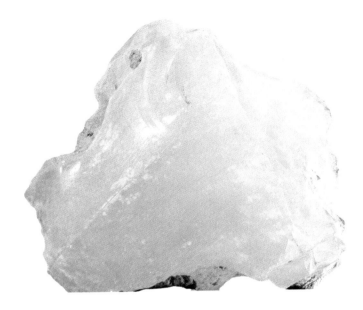

WE SUPPORT A HEALTHY "SELF LOVE FIRST" ATTITUDE.
WE MODEL 7 ESSENTIALS OF SELF-ESTEEM.

1. SELF-ACCOUNTABILITY
2. SELF-AWARENESS
3. SELF-CONFIDENCE
4. SELF-CONTROL
5. SELF-ENCOURAGEMENT
6. SELF-IMPROVEMENT
7. SELF-WORTH

SELF-ESTEEM

ARE YOU A RISK TAKER?
IMAGINE POSSIBLE <u>POSITIVE</u>
OUTCOMES TO A RISK NOT YET
TAKEN.

WILL YOU TAKE THE RISK?

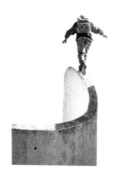

HEALTH-CONSCIOUS

ON DAYS THAT I FEEL AMAZING
PHYSICALLY I'VE NOTICED:

ON DAYS THAT I DON'T FEEL MY
BEST PHYSICALLY I'VE NOTICED:

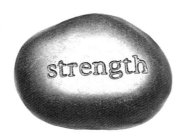

REST
&
RECREATION

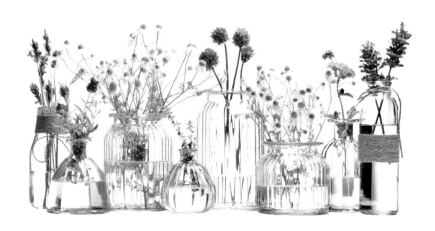

INTELLECT-DEVELOPMENT

```
A  E  P  Y  L  A  N  G  Y  L  A  N  G  Y  L  G
V  I  W  A  V  W  I  H  I  R  B  P  E  L  C  C
P  P  T  S  T  Z  P  Y  I  Q  K  V  I  E  A  I
T  L  C  O  L  C  D  M  K  K  E  H  Q  L  R  A
O  V  T  O  O  L  H  M  M  L  V  L  O  D  D  C
M  W  X  I  D  R  T  O  T  T  Q  O  C  E  A  V
A  G  A  X  I  G  A  R  U  T  C  A  R  E  M  A
G  Q  V  H  I  L  Y  C  E  L  M  T  T  N  O  N
R  K  F  Y  D  M  I  G  I  K  I  D  C  R  M  I
E  W  H  K  I  B  Q  X  U  L  K  D  F  I  B  L
B  C  L  A  R  Y  S  A  G  E  E  R  J  F  C  L
C  Z  H  A  J  Z  U  B  W  Z  N  G  K  F  A  A
E  P  E  T  I  T  G  R  A  I  N  G  N  M  H  U
T  R  D  N  A  B  P  W  L  Z  Y  M  F  A  M  L
J  S  J  X  B  U  C  Y  K  P  T  G  Q  K  E  Y
C  W  W  F  H  S  Y  W  N  A  Q  Y  J  J  Q  U
```

- Angelica Root
- Ylang Ylang
- Clary Sage
- Fir Needle
- Petitgrain
- Patchouli
- Bergamot
- Cardamom
- Vanilla
- Myrtle

AROMAS

NUTRITIONAL-VALUE

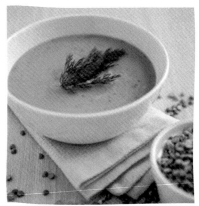

VEGAN SPLIT PEA SOUP

DESCRIPTION
THIS SOUP IS FLAVORFUL AND HEARTY. IT IS ALSO LOW CALORIE.

PREP TIME: 10 MINUTES
COOK TIME: 4 HOURS
TOTAL TIME: 4 HOURS 10 MINUTES
SERVINGS: 8

NUTRITION FACTS
PER SERVING
CALORIES: 149
FAT: 1G
CARBOHYDRATE: 30G
PROTEIN: 7G

INGREDIENTS

2 CUPS OF GREEN SPLIT PEAS, UNCOOKED
8 CUPS OF VEGETABLE BROTH, OR WATER
2 CUBES OF VEGETARIAN BOUILLON
2 MEDIUM POTATOES, CHOPPED
OPTIONAL: 2 RIBS OF CELERY, CHOPPED
2 LARGE CARROTS, SLICED
1 ONION, DICED
2 CLOVES OF GARLIC, MINCED
1 TEASPOON OF DRY MUSTARD
1 TEASPOON OF CUMIN
1 TEASPOON OF SAGE
1 TEASPOON OF THYME
3 LARGE BAY LEAVES

INSTRUCTIONS
1. PUT THE VEGETABLE BROTH, SPLIT PEAS, AND BOUILLON CUBES IN THE SLOW COOKER AND STIR TO COMBINE. ADD THE CELERY, CHOPPED POTATOES, CARROTS, GARLIC, AND ONION.
2. ADD THE CUMIN, MUSTARD, THYME, SAGE, AND BAY LEAVES. STIR THE MIXTURE TO MIX. SEASON WITH PEPPER AND SALT.
3. COVER THE SLOW COOKER AND COOK AT LOW SETTING UNTIL THE GREEN SPLIT PEAS ARE SOFT, ABOUT FOUR HOURS.
4. TASTE AND ADJUST SEASONING IF DESIRED. (REMOVE BAY LEAVES)
5. SERVE.

EXERCISE-PRACTICE

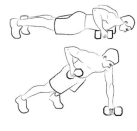

RENEGADE PUSH-UPS!
1. STARTING IN THE PUSHUP POSITION WITH A DUMBBELL IN EACH HAND PERFORM A SINGLE PUSHUP THEN REST IN THE UP POSITION
2. BALANCE YOUR WEIGHT ONTO YOUR RIGHT SIDE AND ROW YOUR LEFT ARM BACKWARDS
3. LOWER YOUR ARM AND REPEAT THE SAME ACTIONS ON THE LEFT SIDE THIS IS 1 REP

BICEP CURLS!
1. STANDING WITH YOUR FEET HIP-WIDTH APART HOLDING A DUMBBELL IN EACH HAND
2. KEEP YOUR ELBOWS CLOSE TO YOUR SIDE AND ROLL YOUR PALMS OUTWARD YOUR FINGERS SHOULD BE FACING FORWARD
3. KEEP YOUR ARMS IN PLACE, BENDING ONLY AT THE ELBOW CURL THE WEIGHTS UP TO YOUR SHOULDERS THEN SLOWLY LOWER THE WEIGHTS AND REPEAT

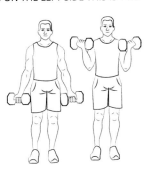
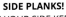

SIDE PLANKS!
1. LAYING ON YOUR SIDE KEEP YOUR FEET TOGETHER AND PLACE YOUR FOREARM DIRECTLY BELOW YOUR SHOULDER
2. FULLY ENGAGE YOUR CORE AND LIFT YOUR HIPS OFF THE FLOOR UNTIL YOUR BODY IS IN A STRAIGHT LINE HOLD HERE FOR ALLOTTED PERIOD
3. RESET AND REPEAT ON THE OTHER SIDE

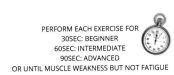

PERFORM EACH EXERCISE FOR
30SEC: BEGINNER
60SEC: INTERMEDIATE
90SEC: ADVANCED
OR UNTIL MUSCLE WEAKNESS BUT NOT FATIGUE

REFLECT
&
RELEASE

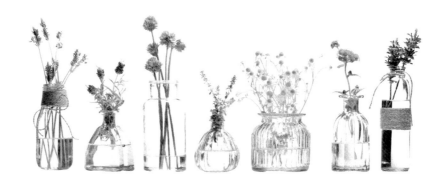

RUBY

ENERGY · LOVE · PASSION

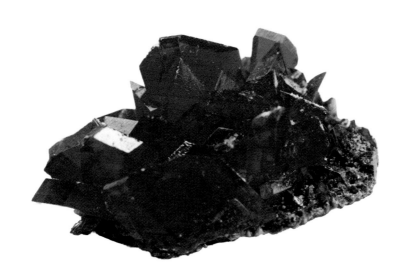

WE PROMOTE AWARENESS OF YOUR CURRENT HEALTH STATUS AND THE INCLUSION OF POSITIVE LIFESTYLE CHANGES TO IMPROVE OVERALL HEALTH.

SELF-ESTEEM

DO YOU HAVE A PLAYLIST THAT
YOU WOULD CONSIDER YOUR
"AUDIO"BIOGRAPHY?

SONG: ARTIST:

SONG: ARTIST:

SONG: ARTIST:

WHAT ARE SOME OF YOUR
FAVORITE LYRICS?

LYRICS:

LYRICS:

LYRICS:

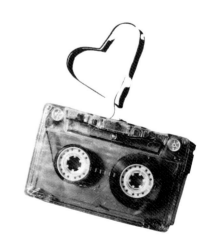

HEALTH-CONSCIOUS

ON DAYS THAT I FEEL AMAZING
MENTALLY I'VE NOTICED:

ON DAYS THAT I DON'T FEEL MY
BEST MENTALLY I'VE NOTICED:

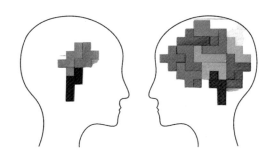

REST
&
RECREATION

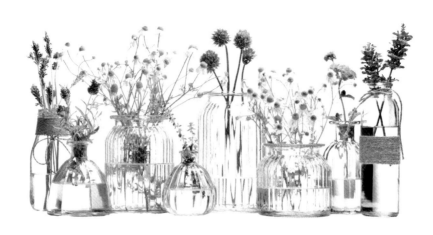

INTELLECT-DEVELOPMENT

```
Z  L  F  F  D  X  E  H  F  A  C  T  E  H  G  E  G
W  A  Z  G  B  B  C  Q  A  E  V  G  J  Y  X  Z  T
Z  O  I  S  I  T  E  S  N  I  K  P  R  H  T  G  H
X  Q  J  W  P  K  X  O  K  B  Z  K  U  R  V  O  A
U  T  I  Z  R  G  T  B  H  P  S  Q  A  Z  I  Z  U
W  B  I  V  R  S  C  V  K  Z  L  U  E  L  M  Q  A
B  V  N  F  N  U  B  C  I  V  Q  U  E  J  S  U  U
S  E  U  O  F  O  B  N  F  Y  R  Y  B  Q  E  A  A
Y  B  O  L  J  A  L  Y  K  N  E  O  C  H  R  R  F
L  M  Y  Y  E  L  N  O  B  S  H  K  N  E  P  T  V
B  J  M  T  M  S  M  Y  R  I  S  U  F  Y  E  Z  Y
A  W  A  Z  P  S  O  E  S  B  P  R  F  V  N  S  J
Y  A  B  F  D  B  G  G  W  T  F  L  E  H  T  D  Q
M  Z  P  G  W  I  Z  F  Q  I  O  B  K  F  I  H  P
Y  H  W  K  T  F  M  X  E  T  T  N  J  K  N  M  R
P  M  R  O  S  E  Q  U  A  R  T  Z  E  O  E  N  B
F  O  H  A  P  R  F  O  P  A  L  Y  W  X  H  P  M
```

- Opal
- Ruby
- Quartz
- Zoisite
- Moonstone
- Tigers Eye
- Rose Quartz
- Serpentine
- Smoky Quartz
- Tiffany Stone

CRYSTALS

NUTRITIONAL-VALUE

INGREDIENTS

1 JULIENNED HEAD OF ROMAINE
LETTUCE
1/2 CUP OF DICED TOMATOES
1/2 CUP OF COOKED
OR CANNED RED BEANS
1/2 CUP OF CHOPPED TEMPEH
BACON
1/2 CUP OF DICED AVOCADO
1/2 CUP OF CORN
1/2 CUP OF RAW
UNSALTED CASHEWS
FOR THE DRESSING:
1/4 CUP OF EXTRA VIRGIN
OLIVE OIL
1/4 CUP OF WATER
1/4 CUP OF AGAVE SYRUP
3 TABLESPOON OF SOY SAUCE
2 TABLESPOONS OF
APPLE CIDER VINEGAR
2 TABLESPOONS OF LEMON JUICE
2 TABLESPOONS OF DIJON
MUSTARD
1 TEASPOON OF GARLIC POWDER

EASY VEGAN COBB SALAD

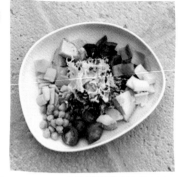

NUTRITION FACTS

PER SERVING
CALORIES: 279
FAT: 3.1G
CARBOHYDRATE:
26.7G
PROTEIN: 8G

DESCRIPTION

THIS IS A HEALTHIER AND
TASTY VERSION OF THE
TRADITIONAL COBB SALAD. IT
IS PACKED WITH NUTRIENTS.
PREP/COOKING TIME: 15
MINUTES
SERVINGS: 6

INSTRUCTIONS

1. PUT THE LETTUCE IN A BOWL
AND TOP WITH ROWS OF RED
BEANS, TOMATOES, TEMPEH,
CORN, AVOCADO, AND
CASHEWS.
2. BLEND ALL THE DRESSING
INGREDIENTS IN A BLENDER
UNTIL SMOOTH. DRIZZLE THE
DRESSING OVER THE SALAD.
3. SERVE.

EXERCISE-PRACTICE

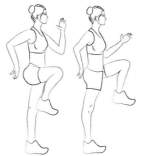

MARCHING STEPS!
1. STANDING WITH YOUR FEET HIP-WIDTH APART
2. BEGIN LIFTING EACH KNEE UP AND DOWN AS IF MARCHING IN PLACE
3. REPEAT MOTION FOR ALLOTTED TIME

MOUNTAIN CLIMBERS!
1. BEGINNING IN THE PUSH-UP POSITION BRING YOUR LEFT FOOT FORWARD TOUCHING YOUR KNEE TO YOUR CHEST KEEPING THE RIGHT LEG EXTENDED
2. HOLDING THAT SAME POSITION QUICKLY SWITCH LEGS
3. REPEAT FOR ALLOTTED TIME

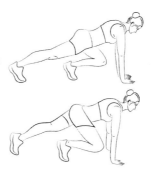

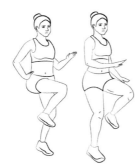

HIGH KNEES!
1. STANDING WITH YOUR FEET HIP-WIDTH APART RAISE YOUR LEFT KNEE TO YOUR CHEST.
2. LOWER THE LEG AND REPEAT ON THE OTHER SIDE
3. KEEPING YOUR CORE TIGHT CONTINUE ALTERNATING LEGS INCREASING SPEED

PERFORM EACH EXERCISE FOR
30SEC: BEGINNER
60SEC: INTERMEDIATE
90SEC: ADVANCED
OR UNTIL MUSCLE WEAKNESS BUT NOT FATIGUE

REFLECT
&
RELEASE

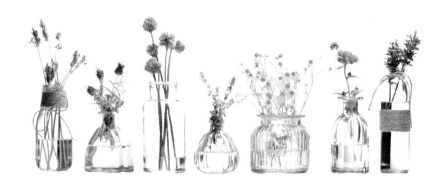

BLUE TOPAZ

CLARITY · FRIENDSHIP · HONESTY

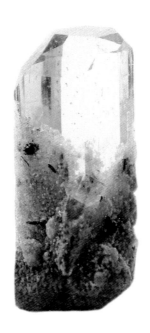

WE ENCOURAGE MENTAL STIMULATION,
THROUGH VARIOUS METHODS OF BRAIN
EXERCISE, CENTERING MENTAL-FOCUS
PRACTICES, AND OTHER STRESS REDUCTION
TECHNIQUES.

SELF-ESTEEM

DO YOU HAVE A SUPPORT
TEAM?

WHAT ARE SOME OF THE
WAYS THAT THEY SUPPORT
YOUR GOALS AND IDEAS?

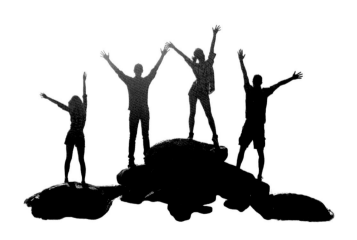

HEALTH-CONSCIOUS

I _____ MY
CURRENT WEIGHT.

I WOULD LIKE TO IMPROVE:

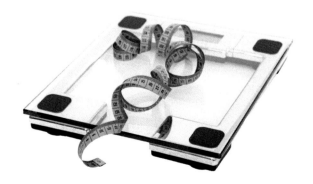

REST
&
RECREATION

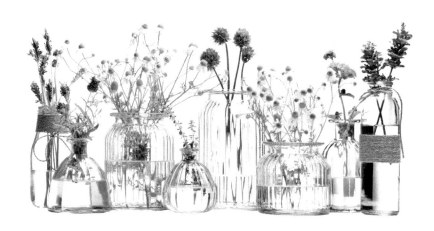

```
T Z Q Z U R X R E D H E K B H Q Q
W P F L E M O T V E L F N K Y G Q
M U P U R Z X D E P M O W O B A S
V I B I Z A M J P J B J E G N U B
S R R Y T P M A S L C L E T L I R
M A Y A H A R B U G P Z Z K W Y E
X R L R C A Y N U P U V H Q Z B A
L Z D M G L P A A T R U Q P Q G D
M B S U O N E R F U A T F G Q Z F
I C S M Z N A F V J D N F K C O R
L P D K L T B Q R H N Q W E T L U
M Z C S S S Z E G U E G U E T F I
F B W M C K L Q R D I F I Z H H T
Z T B V C U T J O R H T X X Z E C
S T A R F R U I T N Y X C I X P N
B A E L A M A E G D I V T Z O F W
Q A V V F O Q Y P W F J M I N O C
```

- BAEL
- NONI
- PITAYA
- RAMBUTAN
- STAR APPLE
- STAR FRUIT
- BREADFRUIT
- SUGAR APPLE
- SALMONBERRY
- MIRACLE FRUIT

EXOTIC FRUITS

NUTRITIONAL-VALUE

INGREDIENTS

1 BANANA (PEELED,
QUARTERED AND
FROZEN)
1/2 CUP OF MIXED
FROZEN BERRIES
1 TABLESPOON OF
FLAXSEED MEAL
1 HEAPING
TABLESPOON OF
SALTED PEANUT
BUTTER
1/2 – 3/4 CUP OF
UNSWEETENED
VANILLA ALMOND
MILK
2 CUPS OF FRESH
SPINACH

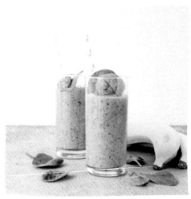

AMAZING GREEN
SMOOTHIE

DESCRIPTION
THIS SMOOTHIE IS SWEET, CREAMY
AND TASTES GREAT. IT'S VERY
HEALTHY AND IT'S GREAT FOR
BREAKFAST OR A MIDDAY SNACK.
PREP/TOTAL TIME: 5 MINUTES
SERVINGS: 1

INSTRUCTIONS
1. ADD ALL THE INGREDIENTS INTO A BLENDER AND PUREE
UNTIL SMOOTH.
2. SERVE.

NUTRITION FACTS
PER SERVING
CALORIES: 314
FAT: 13.4
CARBOHYDRATE: 44.2G
PROTEIN: 10G

EXERCISE-PRACTICE

SIDE LEG RAISES!
1. STANDING WITH YOUR FEET HIP-WIDTH APART
2. LIFT YOUR LEFT LEG OUT TO THE SIDE (TIP: YOU CAN HOLD ONTO SOMETHING STATIONARY FOR BALANCE)
3. HOLD THIS POSITION FOR 1 SECOND THEN SLOWLY LOWER YOUR LEG.
4. SWITCH SIDE AND REPEAT

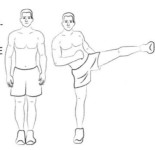

FORWARD LUNGES!
1. STANDING WITH YOUR FEET HIP-WIDTH APART HOLD A DUMBBELL IN EACH HAND AND TAKE A LARGE STEP BACKWARD
2. BEND YOUR FRONT KNEE TO A 90-DEGREE ANGLE ALLOWING THE BACK KNEE TO SLIGHTLY TOUCH THE FLOOR KEEPING YOUR UPPER BODY STRAIGHT
3. PUSH YOUR FRONT HEEL INTO THE FLOOR TO RETURN TO STANDING THEN REPEAT ON THE OTHER SIDE

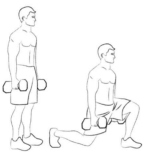

GOBLET SQUATS!
1. STANDING WITH YOUR FEET HIP-WIDTH APART HOLDING A DUMBBELL VERTICALLY BY ONE END
2. KEEPING YOUR UPPER BODY STIFF AND YOUR ELBOWS TUCKED IN LOWER YOUR BODY INTO A SQUAT POSITION
3. RETURN TO A STANDING POSITION AND REPEAT

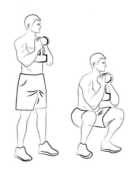

PERFORM EACH EXERCISE FOR
30SEC: BEGINNER
60SEC: INTERMEDIATE
90SEC: ADVANCED
OR UNTIL MUSCLE WEAKNESS BUT NOT FATIGUE

REFLECT
&
RELEASE

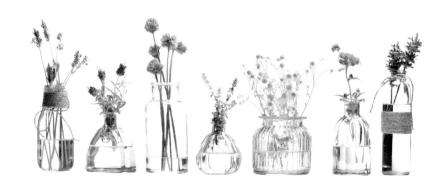

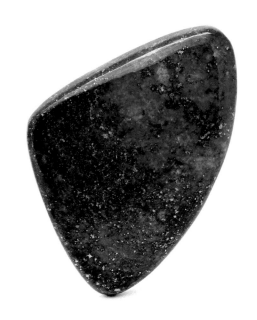

WE BELIEVE IN MAKING THE RIGHT FOOD CHOICES
FOR YOUR BODY WITH THE GOAL OF IMPROVED
HEALTH, AND MAINTAINING A HEALTHY WEIGHT.
WE FOLLOW THE RECOMMENDATIONS LISTED IN
THE DIETARY GUIDELINES FOR AMERICANS.

SELF-ESTEEM

IS THERE A BOOK OR MOVIE THAT
HAS MOTIVATED YOU TO CHANGE
FOR THE BETTER?

WHAT ACTIONS HAVE YOU TAKEN
TO EMBRACE THE CHANGE?

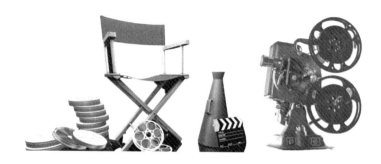

HEALTH-CONSCIOUS

I _____ MY DIETARY CHOICES.

I WOULD LIKE TO IMPROVE:

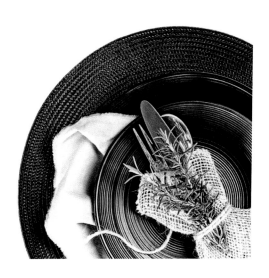

REST
&
RECREATION

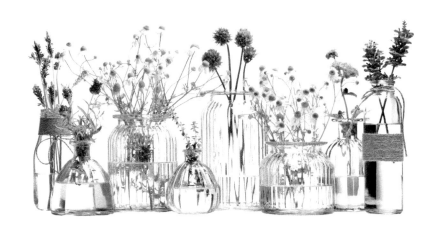

```
A  N  M  R  U  G  E  X  G  B  R  D  O  P  Z  C  T  C
D  J  T  O  T  H  H  Y  R  F  A  G  J  E  E  S  B  H
K  C  Y  Z  Y  Y  X  F  R  P  F  K  U  U  P  T  B  R
G  Z  H  Z  E  B  C  O  R  D  I  E  R  I  T  E  Z  Y
Y  R  U  R  S  K  V  H  L  J  K  H  L  T  A  B  C  S
R  D  B  E  Y  X  R  D  G  H  Q  S  Z  C  L  O  G  O
V  A  X  Z  H  S  A  N  D  A  L  U  S  I  T  E  J  B
H  P  G  Y  W  V  O  H  O  G  D  H  Q  X  K  E  O  E
V  S  C  O  Y  A  S  P  Z  F  K  U  P  F  N  I  C  R
Q  I  Y  Q  L  J  N  E  R  P  Y  O  L  I  Q  K  J  Y
B  U  X  J  O  D  T  Y  G  A  G  O  R  B  X  P  C  L
V  K  S  M  P  I  S  U  O  G  S  T  C  G  L  B  Q  Z
S  M  E  G  L  R  P  T  Q  L  E  E  I  E  R  O  C  B
H  L  S  O  A  N  F  L  O  M  I  I  Q  O  R  D  J  X
Y  I  M  C  B  F  N  Z  A  N  Z  T  Q  D  O  L  Q  A
W  M  P  X  J  V  P  I  V  Q  E  P  E  E  J  Y  D  U
A  V  V  S  I  O  K  M  P  Q  W  V  J  S  P  V  D  Q
D  T  Z  J  G  O  G  E  M  S  I  L  I  C  A  J  W  D
```

- Ametrine
- Ammolite
- Andalusite
- Anyolite
- Chrysoberyl
- Chrysoprase
- Cordierite
- Gem Silica
- Geodes
- Goldstone

CRYSTALS

CREAMY VEGAN PUMPKIN SOUP

<u>INGREDIENTS</u>

1 TABLESPOON OF
VEGAN BUTTER
1 MEDIUM ONION,
DICED
1 CAN OF PUMPKIN
PUREE(16-OUNCE)
1 1/3 CUPS OF
VEGETABLE BROTH
3 CUPS OF SOY
MILK
1/2 TEASPOON OF
NUTMEG
1/2 TEASPOON OF
SUGAR
PEPPER AND SALT

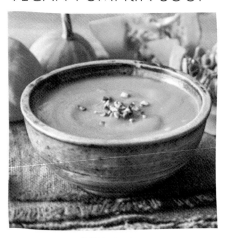

<u>DESCRIPTION</u>
THIS SOUP IS VERY FILLING AND VERY QUICK
TO MAKE. IT'S A SAVORY HOMEMADE SOUP
PREP TIME: 10 MINUTES
COOK TIME: 15 MINUTES
TOTAL TIME: 25 MINUTES
SERVINGS: 4

<u>INSTRUCTIONS</u>

1. COOK THE ONION IN THE BUTTER IN A SAUCEPAN PLACED
OVER MEDIUM HEAT FOR ABOUT FIVE MINUTES. THEN ADD IN
THE REST OF THE INGREDIENTS AND STIR TO MIX.
2. COOK FOR AN ADDITIONAL FIFTEEN MINUTES ON LOW
STIRRING OCCASIONALLY.
3. SERVE.

<u>NUTRITION FACTS</u>
PER SERVING
CALORIES: 148
FAT: 3G
CARBOHYDRATE: 25G
PROTEIN: 5G

EXERCISE-PRACTICE

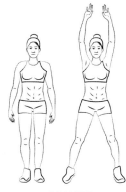

JUMPING JACKS!
1. STANDING WITH YOUR FEET HIP-WIDTH APART AND YOUR ARMS AT YOUR SIDES BEND YOUR KNEES SLIGHTLY, AND JUMP INTO THE AIR
2. WHILE IN THE AIR SPREAD YOUR LEGS SHOULDER-WIDTH APART AND STRETCH YOUR ARMS WING-STYLE OVER YOUR HEAD
3. JUMP BACK INTO THE STARTING POSITION AND REPEAT STEPS 1 AND 2

BURPEES!
1. STARTING IN A DEEP SQUAT POSITION WITH YOUR HANDS ON THE FLOOR KICK YOUR FEET BACK INTO A PUSH-UP POSITION
2. COMPLETE A SINGLE PUSH-UP AND QUICKLY RETURN TO YOUR FEET IN THE SQUAT POSITION
3. THEN SPRING UP INTO A JUMP AS HIGH AS POSSIBLE
4. RESET AND REPEAT

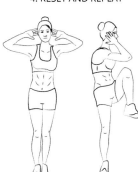

KNEES-TO-ELBOWS!
1. STANDING WITH YOUR FEET HIP-WIDTH APART PLACE YOUR HANDS ON THE SIDE OF YOUR HEAD WITH YOUR ELBOWS POINTED OUTWARD
2. PULL YOUR LEFT LEG UPWARD WHILE TWISTING YOUR TORSO BRING YOUR RIGHT ELBOW TOWARDS YOUR LEFT KNEE
3. RESET AND REPEAT THIS MOVE ALTERNATING SIDES

PERFORM EACH EXERCISE FOR
30SEC: BEGINNER
60SEC: INTERMEDIATE
90SEC: ADVANCED
OR UNTIL MUSCLE WEAKNESS BUT NOT FATIGUE

REFLECT
&
RELEASE

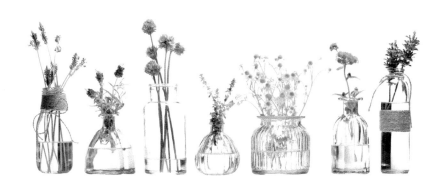

MALACHITE

ABUNDANCE · EMPATHY · WILLPOWER

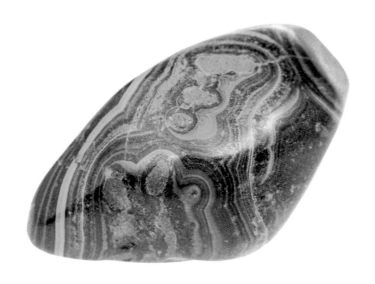

OUR EXERCISE ROUTINES ARE ESPECIALLY DESIGNED TO BE PERFORMED AT EACH PARTICIPANTS UNIQUE ENERGY LEVEL. OUR :30 :60 :90 SECOND COUNTDOWN STYLE ROUTINES ASSIST IN IMPROVING ENDURANCE, STAMINA, AND STRENGTH.

WHAT ARE <u>10</u> AMAZING
TRUTHS ABOUT YOUR
PERSONALITY, THAT EVEN YOU
TAKE FOR GRANTED?

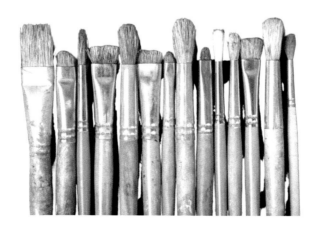

HEALTH-CONSCIOUS

I _____ MY CURRENT
EXERCISE PROGRAM.

I WOULD LIKE TO INCLUDE:

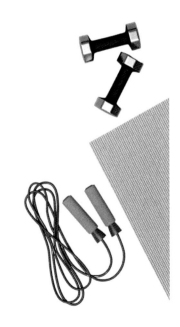

REST
&
RECREATION

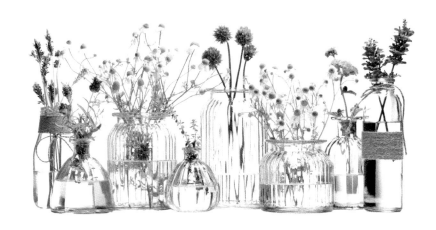

```
K  Q  F  O  R  E  S  T  S  D  R  A  S  P  V  Q
G  F  N  T  W  H  K  Y  O  J  Q  P  U  G  B  U
H  I  K  I  N  G  T  R  A  I  L  S  F  P  S  S
A  X  M  O  X  W  M  C  B  G  P  K  G  K  T  C
T  U  W  P  V  O  H  O  V  E  N  R  C  U  Z  I
J  W  Z  U  A  K  P  N  U  Q  A  A  U  O  V  T
J  A  C  J  S  S  Z  E  K  N  R  C  C  K  W  Y
G  O  A  X  W  M  T  R  N  T  T  Z  H  S  V  S
T  K  J  F  N  V  K  U  L  F  B  A  V  E  P  T
F  F  P  A  R  K  S  O  R  S  I  I  I  F  S  R
K  X  B  Z  X  I  O  P  Q  E  U  E  G  N  L  E
O  T  O  B  I  H  N  U  F  S  S  M  L  O  S  E
C  S  S  H  C  A  D  I  R  T  R  O  A  D  S  T
F  T  L  S  F  I  G  R  S  E  O  T  F  I  S  S
K  Q  F  U  V  X  P  S  P  U  V  W  I  V  N  G
U  N  W  Y  K  Y  L  N  J  D  Z  G  U  P  D  T
```

PARKS	DIRT ROADS	CITY STREETS
BEACHES	MOUNTAINS	HIKING TRAILS
FORESTS	OPEN FIELDS	SCHOOL TRACKS
PASTURES		

OUTDOOR ADVENTURES

NUTRITIONAL-VALUE

TASTY POTATO SALAD

INGREDIENTS

14 OZ OF POTATOES
½ MEDIUM ONION
12 FRESH CHERRY
TOMATOES
1/2 CUP OF CORN
KERNELS
12 FRESH GREEN
OLIVES
SOME VEGAN
RANCH DRESSING

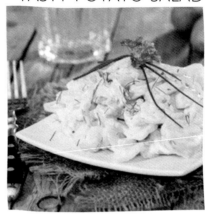

DESCRIPTION
THIS IS MY NEW FAVORITE SALAD. IT TASTES SO GOOD.
PREP TIME: 10 MINUTES
COOK TIME: 20 MINUTES
TOTAL TIME: 30 MINUTES
SERVINGS: 2

INSTRUCTIONS
1. FIRST, COOK THE POTATOES UNTIL SOFT, ABOUT
TWENTY MINUTES. WHEN COOKED, SET ASIDE TO COOL.
CHOP AND TRANSFER THE POTATOES
TO A BOWL.
2. ADD IN THE CHERRY TOMATOES, CHOPPED ONIONS,
GREEN OLIVES, AND CORN KERNELS. ADD THE VEGAN RANCH
DRESSING AND CHILL THE
SALAD IN THE FRIDGE FOR ABOUT TWO HOURS.

NUTRITION FACT
PER SERVING
CALORIES: 256
FAT: 3.5G
CARBOHYDRATE: 51.4G
PROTEIN: 6.8G

EXERCISE-PRACTICE

LUNGES W/ BICEP CURLS!
1: STANDING WITH YOUR FEET HIP-WIDTH
APART HOLD A DUMBBELL IN EACH HAND
AND TAKE A LARGE STEP BACKWARD
2: BRING THE WEIGHTS IN TOWARDS
YOUR SHOULDERS TO COMPLETE A BICEP
CURL
3: PUSH OFF ON THE FRONT FOOT TO
RETURN TO STANDING
4: RESET AND REPEAT

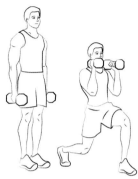

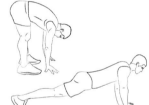

PLANK WALKOUT!
1: STANDING WITH YOUR FEET HIP-WIDTH APART
BRING YOUR HANDS TO THE FLOOR BENDING
THE KNEES IF NECESSARY
2: KEEPING YOUR CORE ENGAGED AND SLOWLY
WALK YOUR HANDS OUT INTO A PLANK KEEPING
YOUR TOES IN PLACE
3: WALK HANDS BACK TO THE STARTING
POSITION AND REPEAT

W-EXTENSIONS!
1: LAYING FACE DOWN WITH YOUR ARMS
BENT AT YOUR SIDE AND YOUR LEGS
FULLY EXTENDED.
2: KEEP YOUR TORSO STABLE AND RAISE
YOUR ARMS AND LEGS TO FORM A SLIGHT
CURVE IN YOUR BODY.
3: RESET AND REPEAT

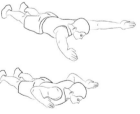

PERFORM EACH EXERCISE FOR
30SEC: BEGINNER
60SEC: INTERMEDIATE
90SEC: ADVANCED
OR UNTIL MUSCLE WEAKNESS BUT NOT FATIGUE

REFLECT
&
RELEASE

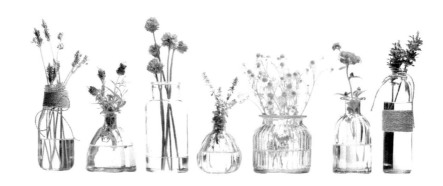

PYRITE

ASSERTIVENESS · PERSISTENCE · VITALITY

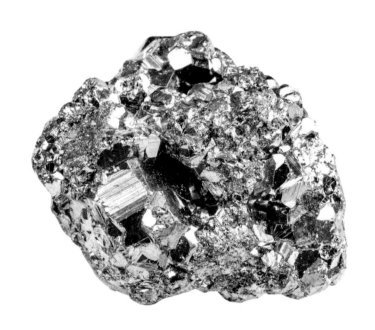

"LIFE IS A FESTIVAL ONLY TO THE WISE."
- RALPH WALDO EMERSON.

SELF-ESTEEM

DO YOU ENGAGE IN POSITIVE
SELF-TALK?

HOW DO YOU COMBAT NEGATIVE
THOUGHTS?

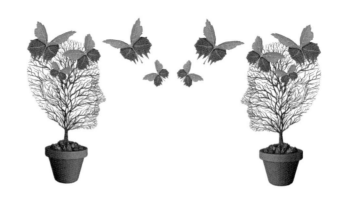

HEALTH-CONSCIOUS

DO YOU SPEND TIME <u>POSITIVELY</u>
ASSESSING THE DAY AHEAD?

WHAT ARE SOME WAYS THAT YOU
PREPARE FOR THE <u>NEXT</u> DAY?

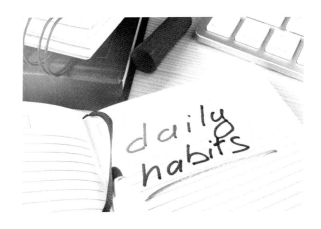

REST
&
RECREATION

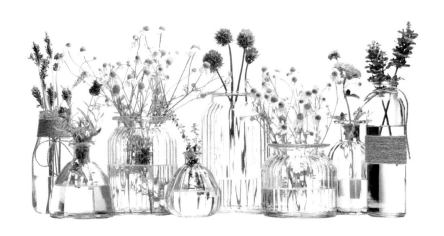

INTELLECT-DEVELOPMENT

```
E  B  U  D  G  V  V  S  M  P  N  F  Z  Z  Q  I  E  T  O
J  P  B  L  A  B  R  A  D  O  R  I  T  E  T  T  E  Z  R
L  A  D  Y  S  S  K  C  D  T  S  U  Z  H  A  F  Q  G  S
V  M  D  M  T  I  O  G  I  T  T  I  E  G  B  G  I  G  C
W  Q  A  E  T  B  E  S  P  W  V  L  A  T  F  P  P  R  N
M  Q  R  Y  N  F  T  B  L  X  M  S  M  D  N  Z  Q  N  S
R  M  I  R  Y  I  J  T  Z  G  S  O  J  A  V  E  D  Z  M
W  L  K  Z  S  X  S  D  T  O  K  M  E  E  T  V  X  B  W
E  C  V  W  A  Y  V  I  M  C  C  W  T  X  I  T  K  S  Z
Z  V  A  J  K  U  D  A  O  N  Z  A  E  X  G  T  Z  L  M
N  M  U  X  M  J  N  Q  D  L  G  T  P  I  E  R  A  I  B
X  N  I  P  F  A  Y  L  R  A  I  D  G  E  Y  E  B  H  S
H  F  N  N  T  G  F  O  S  V  S  T  S  W  C  E  K  V  A
Y  Z  X  N  C  S  O  I  A  V  Z  Z  E  Q  G  A  X  V  W
R  Z  O  G  X  Y  R  D  R  W  P  V  P  J  I  G  X  I  M
Z  M  I  O  L  I  L  X  S  N  X  Z  L  P  U  A  G  O  I
V  U  T  Z  V  O  B  O  G  U  P  L  G  K  L  T  B  N  Z
I  R  M  H  M  H  Y  K  Y  A  N  I  T  E  N  E  O  M  C
B  C  B  O  H  F  J  Z  F  Y  S  D  M  E  E  L  M  B  C
```

- Iolite
- Iris Agate
- Jade
- Jet
- Kyanite
- Labradorite
- Maw Sit Sit
- Moldavite
- Montana Moss Agate
- Tree Agate

CRYSTALS

NUTRITIONAL-VALUE

INGREDIENTS

1 CUP OF FROZEN
STRAWBERRIES
1 CUP OF CHOPPED
FRESH PINEAPPLE
⅓ CUP OF CHILLED
UNSWEETENED
ALMOND MILK, MORE
IF DESIRED
1 TABLESPOON OF
ALMOND BUTTER

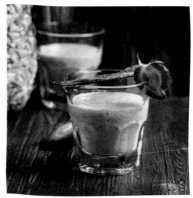

SPARKLING STRAWBERRY SMOOTHIE

DESCRIPTION

THIS IS A DELICIOUS RICH SMOOTHIE. IT'S EASY TO MAKE
AND IT'S READY IN NO TIME.
PREP/TOTAL TIME: 5 MINUTES
SERVINGS: 1

INSTRUCTIONS

1. ADD ALL THE INGREDIENTS INTO A BLENDER AND PUREE
UNTIL SMOOTH.
2. SERVE.

NUTRITION FACTS
PER SERVING:
CALORIES: 255
FAT: 11.1G
CARBOHYDRATE: 39G
PROTEIN: 5.6G

EXERCISE-PRACTICE

ELBOW PLANK!
1: BEGIN IN A MODIFIED PUSHUP POSITION WHERE YOUR WEIGHT IS SUPPORTED BY YOUR FOREARMS AND TOES
2: KEEP YOUR ELBOWS DIRECTLY UNDER YOUR SHOULDERS AND FORM A STRAIGHT LINE FROM YOUR NECK TO YOUR ANKLES
3: FULLY ENGAGE YOUR CORE WHILE HOLDING THE POSITION

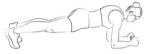

RAISED LEG PLANK!
1: BEGIN IN A MODIFIED PUSHUP POSITION WHERE YOUR WEIGHT IS SUPPORTED BY YOUR FOREARMS AND TOES
2: KEEP YOUR ELBOWS DIRECTLY UNDER YOUR SHOULDERS AND FORM A STRAIGHT LINE FROM YOUR NECK TO YOUR ANKLES
3: ENGAGE YOUR CORE WHILE LIFTING ONE FOOT AT A TIME OFF THE FLOOR

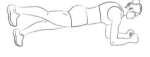

SIDE PLANKS!
1: LAYING ON YOUR LEFT SIDE KEEP YOUR FEET TOGETHER PLACE YOUR LEFT FOREARM DIRECTLY BELOW YOUR SHOULDER
2: FULLY ENGAGE YOUR CORE LIFTING YOUR HIPS OFF THE FLOOR UNTIL YOUR BODY IS IN A STRAIGHT LINE HOLD FOR THE ALLOTTED TIME
3: RESET AND REPEAT ON THE RIGHT SIDE

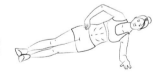

PERFORM EACH EXERCISE FOR
30SEC: BEGINNER
60SEC: INTERMEDIATE
90SEC: ADVANCED
OR UNTIL MUSCLE WEAKNESS BUT NOT FATIGUE

REFLECT
&
RELEASE

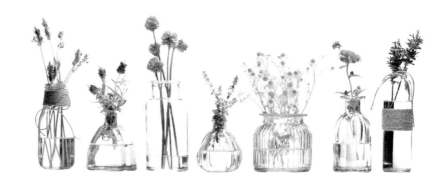

Brecciated Jasper

COMPASSION · GROUNDING · MENTAL FOCUS

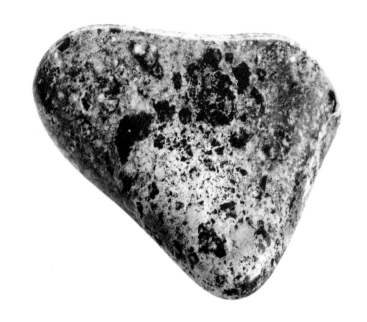

"WHATEVER YOU ARE, BE A GOOD ONE."
-ABRAHAM LINCOLN,

WHAT ARE SOME <u>DAILY</u>
CHALLENGES THAT YOU FACE?

HOW DO YOU <u>OVERCOME</u>
THEM?

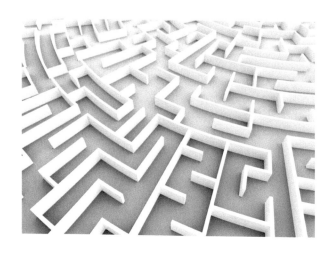

HEALTH-CONSCIOUS

DOES YOUR DAILY ROUTINE
SERVE YOUR BEST INTEREST
HEALTH-WISE?
PLEASE EXPLAIN:

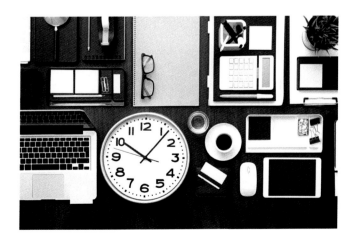

REST
&
RECREATION

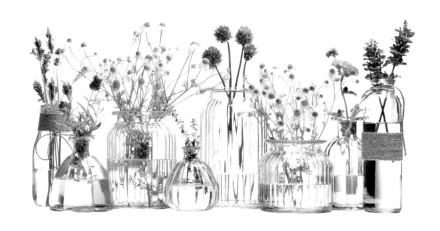

INTELLECT-DEVELOPMENT

```
V  N  E  C  V  H  P  G  L  G  Y  G  N  T  M  K
X  S  S  Y  C  U  O  H  E  T  S  O  Y  D  B  T
G  H  Y  G  I  E  N  E  I  N  I  Z  E  B  W  S
F  W  A  I  J  P  D  L  O  T  E  S  M  O  E  C
E  S  Z  C  T  B  I  I  A  G  C  T  U  P  A  F
S  Z  L  M  T  B  S  L  X  I  A  B  I  H  B  Y
H  C  L  I  I  I  U  B  M  I  F  R  Z  C  Q  N
H  X  W  X  C  C  V  O  Y  W  O  E  I  B  S  D
V  J  E  E  R  L  N  I  J  O  V  A  N  B  U  B
G  L  D  I  L  O  N  O  T  Z  S  T  X  S  M  E
F  A  C  A  G  L  R  G  Q  Y  J  H  X  M  B  Q
H  F  R  R  G  H  N  Z  F  G  K  I  P  Y  M  S
T  O  E  J  E  O  O  E  C  N  E  N  Q  T  O  M
N  A  O  N  R  U  L  P  S  I  F  G  D  D  H  L
T  C  Y  H  Y  U  M  V  F  S  D  U  U  A  J  L
V  E  O  U  X  P  F  Z  V  Q  B  B  V  D  M  E
```

- Circulation
- Flexibility
- Ergonomics
- Breathing
- Decisions
- Activity
- Genetics
- Wellness
- Hygiene

HEALTH IS WEALTH

NUTRITIONAL-VALUE

INGREDIENTS

3/4 POUND OF FRESH
MUSHROOMS, SLICED
1/2 WHITE OR YELLOW
ONION, DICED
2 CLOVES OF GARLIC,
MINCED
1 TABLESPOON OF
VEGAN MARGARINE
3 CUPS OF VEGETABLE
BROTH
2 TABLESPOONS OF
FLOUR
1 CUP OF VEGAN NON-
DAIRY SOUR CREAM
SUBSTITUTE
1 CUP OF SOY MILK

VEGAN CREAM OF MUSHROOM SOUP

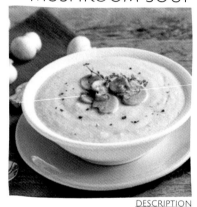

DESCRIPTION
THIS IS A LIGHT AND CREAMY SOUP.
PREP/TOTAL TIME: FIVE MINUTES
SERVINGS: 1

INSTRUCTIONS

1. MELT THE VEGAN MARGARINE IN A POT. ADD IN THE
ONION, MUSHROOMS, AND GARLIC AND COOK OVER
MEDIUM HEAT UNTIL ONIONS SOFTEN, ABOUT FIVE
MINUTES.
2. DECREASE THE HEAT TO LOW AND ADD IN THE
VEGETABLE BROTH. COVER THE POT AND LET IT SIMMER
FOR ABOUT FORTY-FIVE MINUTES.
3. ADD IN THE FLOUR, SOY MILK, AND NON-DAIRY SOUR
CREAM AND STIR TO MIX. LET IT SIMMER ON LOW FOR
ADDITIONAL 10-15 MINUTES TO THICKEN THE SOUP.
4. SEASON THE SOUP WITH PEPPER AND SALT TO TASTE.

NUTRITION FACTS
PER SERVING:
CALORIES: 255
FAT: 11.1G
CARBOHYDRATE: 39G
PROTEIN: 5.6G

EXERCISE-PRACTICE

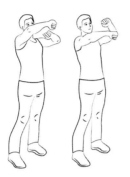

SPEED BAG!
1: HOLDING YOUR FISTS AT CHIN-LEVEL RAISE YOUR ELBOWS UNTIL THEY ARE PARALLEL TO THE FLOOR
2: MAKE SMALL CIRCLES WITH YOUR FISTS AS IF YOU WERE HITTING A SPEED BAG
3: REVERSE THE MOVEMENT, GOING COUNTERCLOCKWISE

ARM CIRCLES!
1: STANDING WITH BOTH ARMS EXTENDING OUTWARD
2: ROTATE ARMS IN A CLOCKWISE DIRECTION FOR THE ALLOTTED TIME
3: RESET AND REVERSE THE MOTION GOING COUNTERCLOCKWISE NEXT

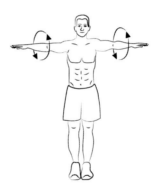

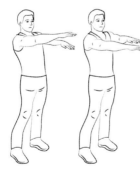

ARM SCISSORS!
1 STANDING WITH BOTH ARMS EXTENDING FRONTWARD
2: QUICKLY OVERLAP YOUR ARMS ALTERNATING LEFT OVER RIGHT AND RIGHT OVER LEFT
3: REPEAT ACTION FOR THE ALLOTTED TIME

PERFORM EACH EXERCISE FOR
30SEC: BEGINNER
60SEC: INTERMEDIATE
90SEC: ADVANCED
OR UNTIL MUSCLE WEAKNESS BUT NOT FATIGUE

REFLECT
&
RELEASE

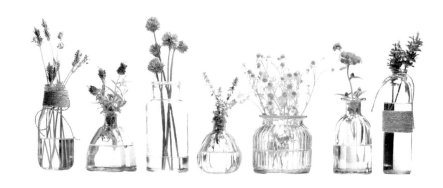

ROSE QUARTZ

HARMONY · LOVE · PEACE

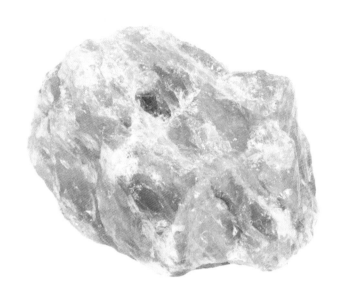

"TRAVEL IS THE FRIVOLOUS PART OF SERIOUS LIVES
AND THE SERIOUS PART OF FRIVOLOUS ONES."
– ANNE SOPHIE SWETCHINE

<u>SELF-ESTEEM</u>

THINK OF SOMEONE YOU HIGHLY RESPECT.

WHAT QUALITIES DO YOU ADMIRE IN THIS PERSON?

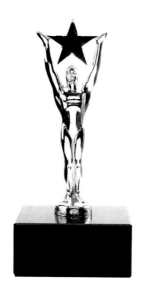

HEALTH-CONSCIOUS

I USE

_____ , _____ , &

_____ ,

TO MANAGE AND COPE WITH

STRESS.

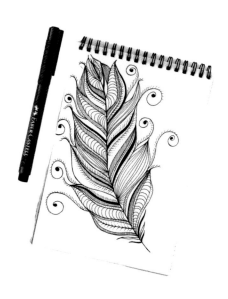

REST
&
RECREATION

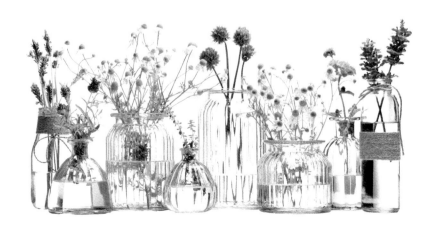

INTELLECT-DEVELOPMENT

```
D R H O D O C H R O S I T E V V F J S
B Z T I I B C I P R M Q O Y Z A J X G
F C S E R I H P P A S Q Z T N G K E M
Q H P I V Z L Z M G S Q A C E P S S R
V G H I R P U A S O N J Y U H I U L P
X F A K H P J H L C T S F I R G G G T
S M L J O Z X B T H A O S N Z Q J I V
Q C E Q D R Q K Z P T P U O X L T B O
E P R T O B C D P F E S O K W M R B G
S G I F N M B H B U A T X L Y J W B V
D D T T I V I V N R O O I O I F F X V
H H E R T R Z J O J Q B D L C T P V K
Q F O L E X X N B M F P H B A L E P R
F P U V M D O S R A S U E B N D D E M
T K E U O S Q U Y P B K F E P H O T F
G L F L Y R E B D E R L F G C K S S W
I F P M A B H M G C F H V H C S N D T
J D E N I T N E P R E S M V F V M N S
Y P Y X J H V Y O X A Z R C R H K F K
```

- Red Beryl
- Sapphire
- Sodalite
- Rhodonite
- Scapolite
- Serpentine
- Sphalerite
- Fancy Sapphire
- Rhodochrosite
- Sonora Sunrise

CRYSTALS

NUTRITIONAL-VALUE

INGREDIENTS

1 CUP OF QUINOA
2 CUPS OF WATER
½ CUP OF CHOPPED
SPRING ONION
1⅓ CUP OF CHOPPED
TOMATOES
1 CUP OF FINELY
CHOPPED FRESH MINT
½ CUP OF FINELY
CHOPPED FRESH
PARSLEY
1 LEMON, JUICED
1 TBS OLIVE OIL

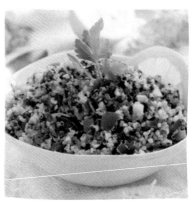

VEGAN QUINOA TABBOULEH

DESCRIPTION
PERFECT SALAD PACKED WITH PROTEIN AND FLAVOR.
PREP/TOTAL TIME: 20 MINUTES
SERVINGS: 2

INSTRUCTIONS

1. FIRST, RINSE THE QUINOA. THEN ADD IN THE
QUINOA INTO BOILING WATER AND LET IT
SIMMER UNTIL ALL WATER HAS BEEN
ABSORBED, ABOUT FIFTEEN MINUTES.
2. WHEN COOKED, SET ASIDE THE QUINOA TO
COOL COMPLETELY. ADD THE QUINOA INTO A
BOWL AND ADD IN THE REMAINING
INGREDIENTS. ADD IN THE OLIVE OIL AND
LEMON JUICE. STIR AND SERVE.

NUTRITION FACTS
CALORIES: 412
FAT: 6.5G
CARBOHYDRATE: 74G
PROTEIN: 17.5G

EXERCISE-PRACTICE

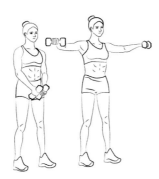

LATERAL RAISES!
1: STANDING WITH YOUR FEET HIP-WIDTH APART HOLD A DUMBBELL IN EACH HAND
2: KEEP YOUR BACK STRAIGHT AND SLOWLY LIFT THE WEIGHTS OUT TO THE SIDE BOTH ARMS SHOULD BE PARALLEL TO THE FLOOR BE SURE TO KEEP YOUR ELBOWS SOMEWHAT BENT
3: LOWER ARMS TO RESET AND REPEAT

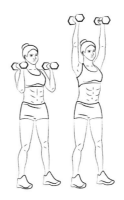

SHOULDER PRESSES!
1: STANDING WITH YOUR FEET HIP-WIDTH APART HOLD A DUMBBELL IN EACH HAND
2: KEEP YOUR BACK STRAIGHT AND SLOWLY LIFT THE WEIGHTS TO THE TOP OF YOUR SHOULDERS THEN PRESS THE WEIGHTS STRAIGHT UPWARDS UNTIL YOUR ARMS ARE DIRECTLY ABOVE YOUR HEAD
3: REVERSE STEPS TO RESET AND REPEAT

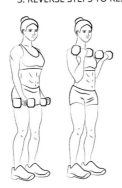

BICEP CURLS!
1. STANDING WITH YOUR FEET HIP-WIDTH APART HOLDING A DUMBBELL IN EACH HAND
2. KEEP YOUR ELBOWS CLOSE TO YOUR SIDE AND ROLL YOUR PALMS OUTWARD YOUR FINGERS SHOULD BE FACING FORWARD
3. KEEP YOUR ARMS IN PLACE BEND AT THE ELBOW CURLING THE WEIGHTS UP TO YOUR SHOULDERS THEN SLOWLY LOWER THE WEIGHTS TO RESET

PERFORM EACH EXERCISE FOR
30SEC: BEGINNER
60SEC: INTERMEDIATE
90SEC: ADVANCED
OR UNTIL MUSCLE WEAKNESS BUT NOT FATIGUE

REFLECT
&
RELEASE

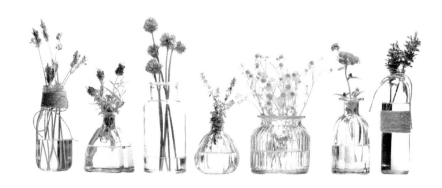

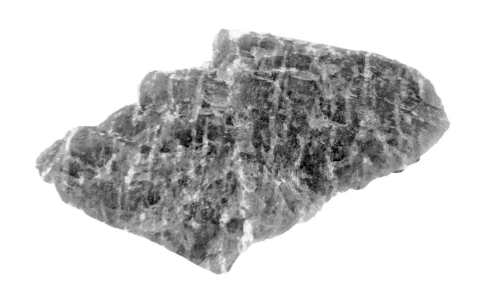

"THE STRONGEST PRINCIPLE OF GROWTH
LIES IN HUMAN CHOICE"
– GEORGE ELIOT

WHAT IS YOUR FAVORITE
MOTIVATIONAL QUOTE?

WHAT DOES IT MEAN TO YOU
IN YOUR WORDS?

HEALTH-CONSCIOUS

I WOULD CLASSIFY MY
SMARTPHONE/SOCIAL MEDIA USAGE AS
_____.

DO YOUR INTERACTIONS INCLUDE
MOSTLY HEALTHY AND POSITIVE
MATERIAL?

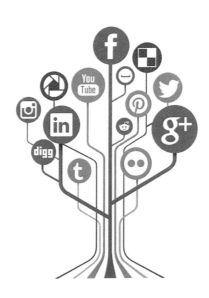

REST
&
RECREATION

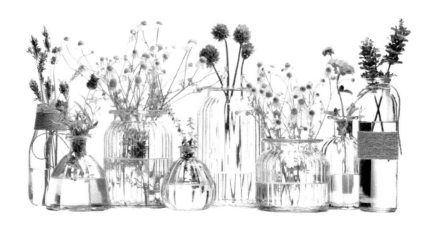

INTELLECT-DEVELOPMENT

```
X  B  S  P  V  U  I  P  N  P  A  U  N  Q
M  O  J  E  O  M  U  S  D  B  M  W  L  U
D  T  Y  R  E  R  V  T  R  W  J  X  W  X
T  S  K  U  J  F  T  U  I  A  B  G  I  Z
Q  W  J  I  D  Z  R  U  K  T  E  A  C  Z
F  A  J  P  O  S  O  W  G  T  A  L  K  V
Z  N  A  B  T  C  N  L  A  A  S  L  F  G
U  A  N  F  C  C  J  S  L  N  L  Z  Y  O
Y  P  A  O  M  E  A  Y  G  E  D  C  I  H
W  T  R  R  N  E  Y  B  U  V  K  A  I  O
V  O  S  O  U  T  H  A  F  R  I  C  A  E
M  C  H  A  R  I  Z  O  N  A  Y  V  S  N
A  R  G  E  N  T  I  N  A  H  I  I  F  N
J  X  V  O  F  D  C  H  X  T  I  N  X  I
```

- Peru
- Italy
- Israel
- Rwanda
- Arizona
- Morocco
- Botswana
- Portugal
- Argentina
- South Africa

VACATION IDEAS

NUTRITIONAL-VALUE

INGREDIENTS

1 LARGE RIPE AVOCADO,
HALVED AND PITTED
1 ½ CUPS OF VANILLA
ALMOND MILK
3 TABLESPOONS OF
UNSWEETENED COCOA
POWDER
3 TABLESPOONS OF
BROWN SUGAR OR
MAPLE SYRUP, OR TO
TASTE
2 TABLESPOONS OF
NONDAIRY SEMISWEET
CHOCOLATE CHIPS,
MELTED
1 TABLESPOON OF
VANILLA EXTRACT, OR
TO TASTE
12 LARGE ICE CUBES

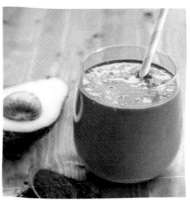

EASY CHOCOLATE AVOCADO SHAKE

DESCRIPTION
THIS SMOOTHIE IS SIMPLY DELICIOUS
YOU WILL ENJOY EVERY SIP.
PREP/TOTAL TIME: 10 MINUTES
SERVINGS: 2

INSTRUCTIONS

1. BLEND THE AVOCADO, COCOA, MILK, BROWN
SUGAR, VANILLA, AND MELTED CHOCOLATE IN
THE BLENDER UNTIL CREAMY AND SMOOTH.
2. ADD IN THE ICE CUBES AND BLEND TO
THICKEN. 3. SERVE.

NUTRITION FACTS
PER SERVING:
CALORIES: 381
FAT: 23.1G
CARBOHYDRATE: 44.8G
PROTEIN: 5.4G

EXERCISE-PRACTICE

BUTT KICKS!
1. STANDING WITH YOUR FEET HIP-WIDTH APART BEND YOUR ARMS AT YOUR SIDES
2. BEND YOUR RIGHT KNEE BACKWARD AND KICK YOUR RIGHT HEEL TOWARD YOUR GLUTES
3. LOWER YOUR RIGHT LEG AND REPEAT ON THE LEFT SIDE INCREASING SPEED

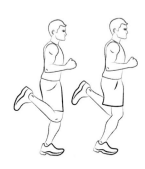

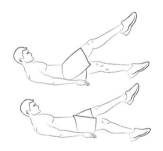

FLUTTER KICKS!
1: START FLAT ON YOUR BACK WITH YOUR ARMS AT YOUR SIDES AND YOUR PALMS FACING DOWN
2: ELEVATE YOUR LEGS 1 TO 6 INCHES OFF THE FLOOR THEN MAKE QUICK UP-AND-DOWN MOVEMENTS WHILE KEEPING YOUR CORE ACTIVATED.
3: CONTINUE FOR THE ALLOTTED TIME

SEAL JACKS!
1: STANDING WITH YOUR FEET HIP-WIDTH APART AND YOUR ARMS AT YOUR SIDES BEND YOUR KNEES SLIGHTLY, AND JUMP INTO THE AIR SPREADING YOUR FEET AND ARMS AT THE SAME TIME.
2: LAND WITH YOUR FEET SPREAD AND THEN IMMEDIATELY JUMP UP AGAIN BRINGING YOUR FEET AND HANDS BACK TOGETHER.
3: RESET AND REPEAT

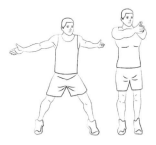

PERFORM EACH EXERCISE FOR
30SEC: BEGINNER
60SEC: INTERMEDIATE
90SEC: ADVANCED
OR UNTIL MUSCLE WEAKNESS BUT NOT FATIGUE

REFLECT
&
RELEASE

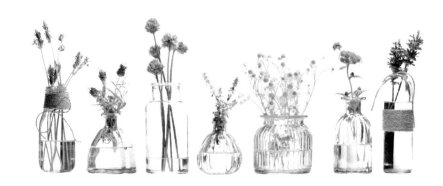

BLUE GOLDSTONE

AMBITION · COURAGE · UPLIFTING

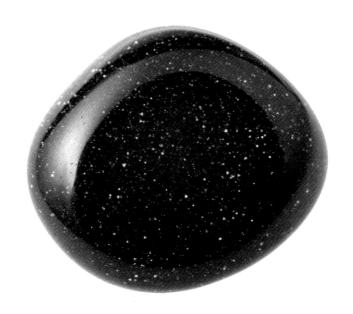

"IF THE WORLD SEEMS COLD TO YOU,
KINDLE FIRES TO WARM IT"
– LUCY LARCOM

SELF-ESTEEM

WHAT ARE YOU
GRATEFUL FOR?

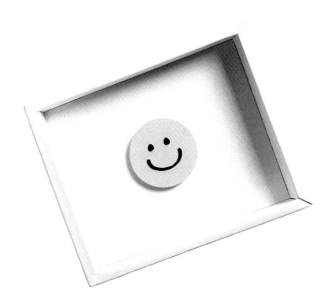

HEALTH-CONSCIOUS

SOME HOLISTIC REMEDIES THAT
I'M FAMILIAR WITH ARE:

I WOULD LIKE TO TRY:

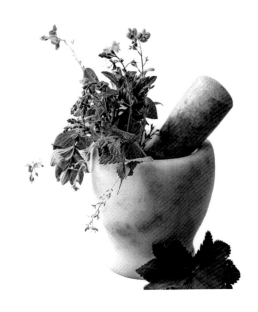

REST
&
RECREATION

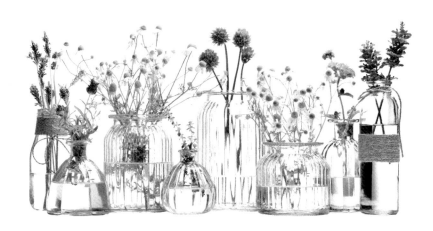

INTELLECT-DEVELOPMENT

```
N  I  N  O  G  K  L  V  H  V  Q  K  H  P  J  P  S
M  G  Q  X  J  G  C  G  M  M  M  T  Q  H  F  T  Y
V  H  F  T  J  B  M  B  C  T  U  Y  R  Z  R  W  L
S  C  B  X  Z  M  L  N  O  R  D  H  F  O  O  F  E
Y  P  B  U  Q  R  C  U  Q  T  X  S  N  R  P  J  N
A  A  H  L  E  K  E  U  E  R  O  T  K  P  Z  P  I
N  T  N  E  X  N  O  S  E  T  I  P  P  O  T  V  P
E  T  W  O  N  I  I  K  P  U  O  Q  A  C  F  V  S
H  T  Z  F  S  E  W  L  M  O  I  P  F  Z  M  V  Z
S  R  I  E  R  I  J  T  A  X  D  K  A  E  V  R  K
E  B  U  N  B  B  I  P  T  M  C  U  G  Z  W  I  J
B  Q  L  P  A  T  U  F  M  G  R  Z  M  J  R  E  L
Q  P  Z  L  A  Z  D  Y  S  B  Z  U  Q  E  M  J  F
B  I  A  N  J  W  N  D  Z  N  C  M  O  S  N  Z  R
Y  H  A  W  C  U  B  A  M  Y  F  K  C  T  T  E  F
J  T  L  H  P  J  R  I  T  M  I  W  Y  B  H  Z  E
E  A  E  N  O  T  S  N  U  S  Y  R  W  C  L  T  K
```

- Sunstone
- Strontium Titanate
- Spodumene
- Turquoise
- Sphene
- Spinel
- Blue Topaz
- Tourmaline
- Topaz
- Tanzanite

CRYSTALS

NUTRITIONAL-VALUE

INGREDIENTS

1 TEASPOON OF OLIVE OIL
1 MEDIUM ONION, DICED
1 MEDIUM CARROT, SLICED
4 CUPS OF VEGETABLE
BROTH
1 CUP OF DRY BROWN
LENTILS
1/4 TEASPOON OF DRIED
THYME
2 LARGE BAY LEAVES
A PINCH OF SALT
PEPPER
OPTIONAL: 2 TEASPOONS
OF LEMON JUICE (IF
DESIRED)

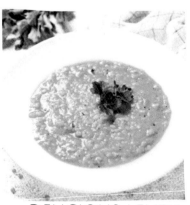

DELICIOUS LENTIL
SOUP

INSTRUCTIONS

1. COOK THE CARROT AND ONIONS IN OLIVE OIL UNTIL
ONIONS TURN CLEAR, ABOUT FIVE MINUTES.
2. ADD IN THE LENTILS, VEGETABLE BROTH, BAY LEAVES,
AND THYME. SEASON WITH PEPPER AND SALT.
3. DECREASE THE HEAT TO A SIMMER, COVER, AND COOK
UNTIL THE LENTILS ARE SOFT, ABOUT FORTY FIVE
MINUTES.
4. REMOVE THE BAY LEAVES AND ADD IN THE LEMON
JUICE IF USING. STIR AND ADJUST SEASON IF DESIRED.
SERVE.

DESCRIPTION
THIS SOUP IS VERY FLAVORFUL AND WARMING
PREP TIME: 5 MINUTES
COOK TIME: 50 MINUTES
TOTAL TIME: 55 MINUTES
SERVINGS: 4

NUTRITION FACTS
CALORIES: 332
FAT: 8G
CARBOHYDRATE: 47G
PROTEIN: 21G

EXERCISE-PRACTICE

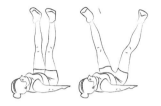

SCISSOR KICKS!
1. START FLAT ON YOUR BACK WITH YOUR ARMS AT YOUR SIDES AND YOUR PALMS FACING DOWN USING YOUR ABS BRING YOUR LEGS STRAIGHT UP
2. OVERLAP YOUR LEGS IN THE CENTER ALTERNATING LEFT OVER RIGHT AND RIGHT OVER LEFT
3. REPEAT ACTION FOR THE ALLOTTED TIME

CALF RAISES!
1. STANDING WITH YOUR FEET HIP-WIDTH APART SLOWLY RISE STRAIGHT UP ON YOUR TOES YOUR HEELS SHOULD LIFT OFF THE FLOOR
2. HOLD FOR A FEW SECONDS THEN LOWER YOUR HEELS BACK DOWN
3. REST AND REPEAT

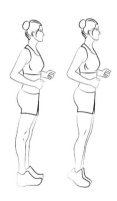

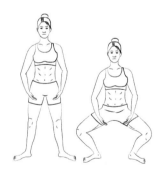

GRAND PLIÉ 2ND POSITION!
1: STANDING WITH YOUR FEET HIP-WIDTH APART TAKE A SHORT STEP OUT TO EITHER SIDE
2: BEND AT THE KNEES AS LOW AS POSSIBLE WHILE HOLDING YOUR SPINE STRAIGHT AND STEADY BE SURE TO KEEP YOUR HEELS ON THE FLOOR
3: EXTEND YOUR LEGS STRAIGHT UP THEN SLOWLY LOWER BACK INTO THE SQUAT POSITION

PERFORM EACH EXERCISE FOR
30SEC: BEGINNER
60SEC: INTERMEDIATE
90SEC: ADVANCED
OR UNTIL MUSCLE WEAKNESS BUT NOT FATIGUE

REFLECT
&
RELEASE

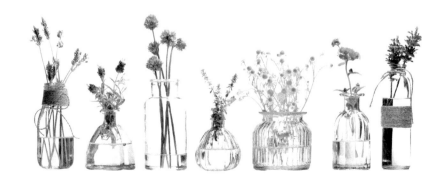

Clear Quartz

CREATIVITY · ENERGY · HEALING

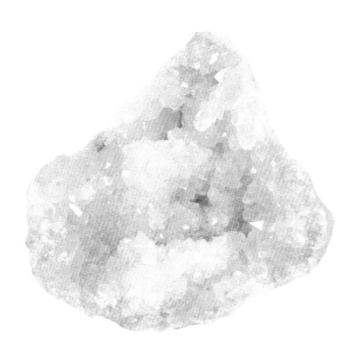

"TO LOVE DEEPLY IN ONE DIRECTION
MAKES US MORE LOVING IN ALL OTHERS"
– ANNE SOPHIE SWETCHINE

SELF-ESTEEM

WHAT <u>VISION</u> DO YOU
HOLD FOR YOUR FUTURE?

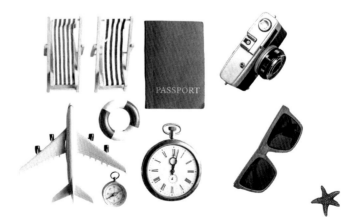

IN THE NEXT 12-WEEKS,
CONCERNING MY HEALTH,
I'D LIKE TO REACH THE
GOAL OF:

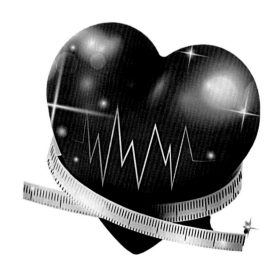

REST
&
RECREATION

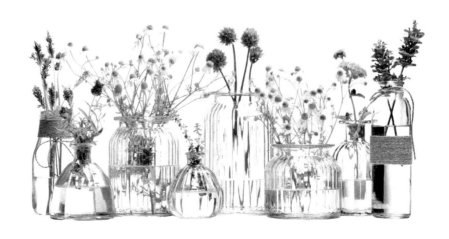

```
C  O  Y  K  T  D  L  Z  U  X  O  I  N  F
F  I  E  U  P  I  T  O  Y  Z  E  J  Y  D
H  F  L  F  S  E  H  P  B  P  X  X  H  P
L  G  E  A  M  N  Y  E  Y  N  O  E  E  F
A  R  B  N  N  R  M  U  X  C  Z  F  C  R
V  G  Y  Q  N  T  E  Z  M  M  J  D  O  V
E  S  G  Z  I  E  R  S  U  Q  I  N  Q  O
N  H  U  R  Y  T  L  O  Z  U  U  N  U  C
D  D  Q  J  C  P  A  R  S  L  E  Y  T  I
E  R  I  C  J  W  I  L  L  E  B  Y  O  C
R  M  V  L  D  Z  O  R  G  H  V  J  K  M
U  N  W  X  L  W  A  A  L  Q  Z  Y  J  T
A  A  R  Y  D  S  S  X  X  S  W  Z  P  M
C  L  C  H  A  M  O  M  I  L  E  J  P  H
```

- Lavender
- Cilantro
- Mint
- Fennel
- Basil
- Dill
- Chamomile
- Thyme
- Sage
- Parsley

HERBS

NUTRITIONAL-VALUE

INGREDIENTS

1 CAN OF SWEET CORN
(15OZ)
1 CAN OF SWEET PEAS
(15OZ)
1 CAN OF CHICKPEAS
(15OZ)
1 CAN OF BLACK BEANS
(15OZ)
½ LARGE ONION, FINELY
CHOPPED
2 CARROTS, GRATED
1/2 CUP OF CILANTRO,
CHOPPED
A PINCH OF SEA SALT
BLACK PEPPER
FRESH LIME JUICE

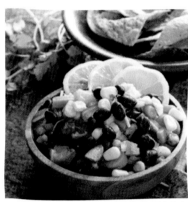

QUICK BLACK BEAN AND CORN SALAD

DESCRIPTION
THIS SALAD IS ENERGIZING AND REFRESHING.
PREP/TOTAL TIME: 10 MINUTES
SERVINGS: 8

INSTRUCTIONS

1. DRAIN THE CANS OF THE BLACK BEANS,
CORN, CHICKPEAS, SWEET PEAS
TRANSFER TO A BOWL AND COMBINE.
2. ADD IN THE CARROTS, RED ONION,
AND CILANTRO. SEASON WITH PEPPER
AND SALT.
3. TOP WITH LIME JUICE. SERVE.

NUTRITION FACTS
PER SERVING
CALORIES: 126
FAT: 15G
CARBOHYDRATE: 24G
PROTEIN: 6G

EXERCISE-PRACTICE

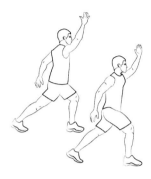

SPLIT JACKS!
1. STAND WITH ONE LEG FORWARD IN A LUNGE POSITION WITH YOUR ARMS DOWN AT YOUR SIDES
2. LEAP INTO THE AIR WHILE SWITCHING LEGS MID-AIR BEFORE LANDING INCORPORATE RAISING THE OPPOSITE ARM TO THE LEADING LEG ON EACH JUMP.
3. CONTINUE FOR THE ALLOTTED TIME

PLANK CRUNCHES!
1. BEGINNING IN THE PUSH-UP POSITION BRING YOUR LEFT FOOT FORWARD TOUCHING YOUR KNEE TO YOUR CHEST KEEPING THE RIGHT LEG EXTENDED
2. KEEPING THE SAME POSITION QUICKLY SWITCH LEGS CRUNCHING THE OBLIQUES
3. REPEAT MOTION FOR ALLOTTED TIME

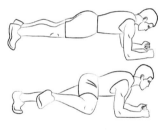

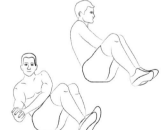

SIT AND TWIST!
1: STARTING IN A SEATED UPRIGHT POSITION KEEP YOUR SHOULDERS BACK AND YOUR CORE FULLY ENGAGED
2: HOLD YOUR HANDS TOGETHER AT WAIST LEVEL TWIST BODY UNTIL THE LEFT ELBOW TOUCHES THE OUTSIDE OF THE RIGHT KNEE
3: ALTERNATE FOR THE ALLOTTED TIME

PERFORM EACH EXERCISE FOR
30SEC: BEGINNER
60SEC: INTERMEDIATE
90SEC: ADVANCED
OR UNTIL MUSCLE WEAKNESS BUT NOT FATIGUE

REWARD YOURSELF!

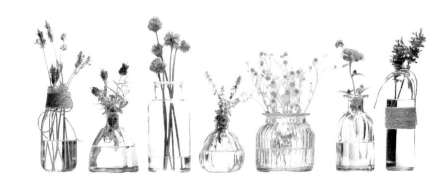

ANSWERS

CRYSTALS

- GARNET
- HEMATITE
- GOLDSTONE
- DIAMOND
- AMAZONITE
- BLOODSTONE
- EMERALD
- FIREAGATE
- LAPISLAZULI
- AMETHYST

AROMAS

- ANGELICAROOT
- PETITGRAIN
- CARDAMOM
- YLANGYLANG
- PATCHOULI
- VANILLA
- CLARYSAGE
- BERGAMOT
- MYRTLE
- FIRNEEDLE

CRYSTALS

- OPAL
- TIGERSEYE
- RUBY
- ROSEQUARTZ
- QUARTZ
- SERPENTINE
- ZOISITE
- SMOKYQUARTZ
- MOONSTONE
- TIFFANYSTONE

EXOTIC FRUITS

- BAEL
- STARAPPLE
- SUGARAPPLE
- NONI
- STARFRUIT
- SALMONBERRY
- PITAYA
- BREADFRUIT
- MIRACLEFRUIT
- RAMBUTAN

CRYSTALS

- AMETRINE
- CHRYSOBERYL
- GEMSILICA
- AMMOLITE
- CHRYSOPRASE
- GEODES
- ANDALUSITE
- CORDIERITE
- GOLDSTONE
- ANYOLITE

OUTDOOR ADVENTURES

- PARKS
- DIRTROADS
- CITYSTREETS
- BEACHES
- MOUNTAINS
- HIKINGTRAILS
- FORESTS
- OPENFIELDS
- SCHOOLTRACKS
- PASTURES

CRYSTALS

- IOLITE
- KYANITE
- MOLDAVITE
- IRISAGATE
- LABRADORITE
- MONTANAMOSSAGATE
- JADE
- MAWSITSIT
- TREEAGATE
- JET

HEALTH IS WEALTH

- CIRCULATION
- BREATHING
- GENETICS
- FLEXIBILITY
- DECISIONS
- WELLNESS
- ERGONOMICS
- ACTIVITY
- HYGIENE

CRYSTALS

- REDBERYL
- SCAPOLITE
- FANCYSAPPHIRE
- SAPPHIRE
- SERPENTINE
- RHODOCHROSITE
- SODALITE
- SPHALERITE
- SONORASUNRISE
- RHODONITE

VACATION IDEAS

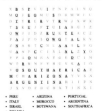

- PERU
- ARIZONA
- PORTUGAL
- ITALY
- MOROCCO
- ARGENTINA
- ISRAEL
- BOTSWANA
- SOUTHAFRICA
- RWANDA

CRYSTALS

- SUNSTONE
- SPHENE
- TOURMALINE
- STRONTIUMTITANATE
- SPINEL
- TOPAZ
- SPODUMENE
- BLUETOPAZ
- TANZANITE
- TURQUOISE

HERBS

- LAVENDER
- BASIL
- THYME
- CILANTRO
- DILL
- SAGE
- MINT
- CHAMOMILE
- PARSLEY
- FENNEL

Gymstones Factory

Know your worth.

ISBN: 978-1-79488-217-1

VISIT:

WWW.GYMSTONESFACTORY.COM

FOR MORE LIFESTYLE AND WEIGHT
MANAGEMENT SOLUTIONS